Bulk Up Like The Hulk

Easy Muscle Mass For Everyone

RON KNESS

ISBN-13: 978-1540658418

ISBN-10: 1540658414

Contents

Disclaimer

This publication is for informational purposes only and is not intended as medical advice. Medical advice should always be obtained from a qualified medical professional for any health conditions or symptoms associated with them.

Every possible effort has been made in preparing and researching this material. We make no warranties with respect to the accuracy, applicability of its contents or any omissions.

See your healthcare professional before starting any diet or exercise program!

Introduction

If you grew up in the late 20th century, who doesn't remember "The Hulk". He was big with a dominating personality. While you may not be able to get as big as the hulk, most people can add mass to their muscles. In this book I delve into the science behind building muscle mass. The process is not that difficult, however it does require a lot of patience and perseverance to become successful. Let's get started ...

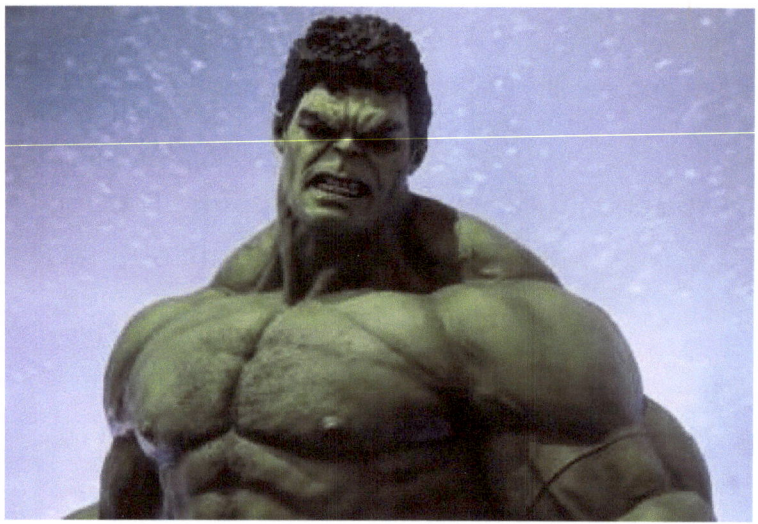

What does it feel like to be jacked? Most that re will tell you in a single word: it feels *incredible*.

Being very strong and taking up a lot of physical space changes the entire way you feel about yourself and the way that others perceive you as well. Suddenly, you become a physical presence and people can't help but sit up and take notice. You become indomitable, immovable and powerful and as a result, everything you say has more weight and more gravity to it.

People *listen*.

Bulking changes other things too. When you feel that powerful and you notice the way people start treating you, you can't help but feel far more confident too. This changes the way you walk, the way you hold yourself and the way that you present yourself. You walk like someone unstoppable and that only increases that sense of presence.

And then there are all the direct and practical ways that gaining muscle changes your life. You start to win play fights with your sparing mates, you become better at sports and people start asking you to help them lift things.

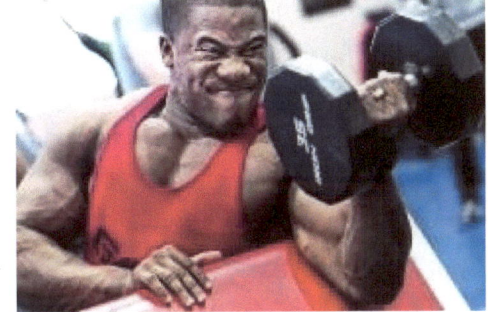

You know, it's just a great feeling to be thought of as someone capable and powerful – instead of being the little guy who is the butt of jokes all the time!

And being jacked also helps you to get attention from the opposite sex. You look amazing in all your clothes – you can fill out a suit and your arms pop from white vests – and all that power and confidence is simply *highly* attractive to people.

You'll even find that you start getting your way more in work and in the rest of your life, as people start to take you more seriously. That, and physical prowess correlates with improved brain power, you can expect to start thinking better too!

But maybe you're not bothered about all that. Maybe you're simply looking for a way to bulk up so you can become stronger and better at your sport. Perhaps you're a bodybuilder?

Whatever the case, this book is going to act as your ultimate guide. Here, you will find everything you could possibly need to know in order to GROW and you'll be given simple, straightforward steps you can follow to do just that.

And the difference this time is that we're going to organize it all in a way that actually *works*. No more half-hearted attempts and no more disappointments. The science is simple, all we have to do is put it into practice...

What You Will Learn

This really is a science and not an art. The way you go about building muscle is *very* simple and once you know the formula, it's a simple matter of following it through to completion. There's no mystery to this formula either – it's something that athletes have been using for decades. All we're going to do that's a bit different, is adapt that bodybuilding formula and make it a little more adaptable so that you can fit it around your busy schedule.

Here's what you will learn, specifically:

- What your genetic potential for gaining muscle is

- How to eat for bulk

- How to fit your eating plan around your lifestyle

- How to eat big while saving money

- The secret to staying (relatively) lean while bulking

- How to increase your strength massively

- The optimum amount of training and way to train for building muscle

- How to dress to look stronger

- How to focus on the muscles that will create the biggest visual impact and strength gains

- How to train and bulk from home

- The best supplements for accelerating growth

- And much more!

Ready to dig deeper into the fascinating world of muscle building ... let's do this!

Chapter 1 – Your Current State

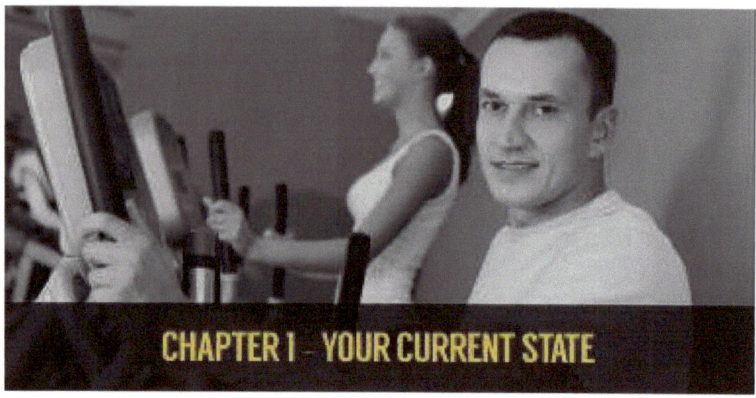

Before we dive into how you're going to bulk, the first thing we need to do is address your current state. That means we'll be looking at your current muscle mass, your height and how much muscle you're likely to gain. We'll also be looking at the metabolic demands of your body, which will tell us how many calories you'll burn in a given day. That's going to be *very* important for building muscle, as we will see in a moment.

So for now, we're going to start by assessing you and your current situation. We'll find some numbers to put to your name and while it might all seem a little random, stick with it. In the chapters that follow, these numbers are going to serve as your guide. Knowing yourself is crucial when it comes to gaining muscle!

So first, let's calculate your current body fat percentage and lean mass...

How to Calculate Your Body Fat Percentage and Lean Mass

Finding out how much you weigh is very easy: all you need to do is step on a set of scales and you'll be given a precise number denoting your weight.

But that on its own is not a particularly useful metric because it doesn't actually tell you anything about your muscle. Anyone can be 'big' – they just have to eat huge amounts of cake! But you're not trying to get fat, you're trying to get *jacked*. That means you're 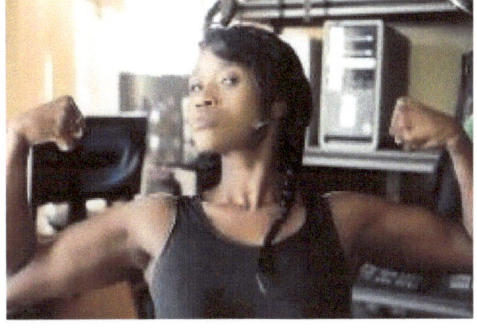 interested in adding muscle and that's why you need to know just how much of your current mass *is* muscle already.

So to do this, you're going to step yourself onto a set of scales and get your weight in lbs. Done that? Let's say you are 176.4 lbs. at 5'8'' for demonstration purposes.

Now, you need to work out your body fat percentage. This is the percentage of that weight that is accounted for by subcutaneous fat (the fat underneath your skin). And finding this number is fortunately very easy – all you need to do is to measure the thickness of your skin which will include that layer of fat.

To do this, you need to grab a pinch of skin from the side of the tricep. So this is the spot mid-way between your shoulder and elbow and on the outside of your arm around from the bicep.

Measure this and then use the chart below to get your current body fat percentage:

Skin fold thickness in mm (inches)	Bodyfat % Men	Bodyfat % women
6 (1/4")	5-9	8-13
13 (1/2")	9-13	13-18
19 (3/4")	13-18	18-23
25 (1")	18-22	23-28
38 (1 ½")	22-27	28-33

This is a rough estimate of course but you can also get an idea by looking at photos of people at different body fat percentages. If you can see abs but aren't covered in ripped veins, then you're probably between 13-10% body fat. If you can see all the striations and the veins, then you're sub 10%.

Find a number that you think is a fair estimate and then subtract that percentage from your current body weight to find out what you would weigh if all of your body fat were to be removed. If you weighed 100lbs and your body fat percentage were 10%, then you would have a lean mass of 90lbs. Let's say that number for you is 158.76lb because you have 10% body fat (approx.).

Calculating Your Genetic Potential

Now it's actually possible to get some more very interesting information from these numbers, which is your FFMI. That's your 'Fat Free Mass Index', which is like a body mass index but a lot more accurate because it differentiates between muscle and fat.

And what's more, is that there is an upper limit to what your FFMI can be naturally without using steroids or other performance enhancing drugs. This is good because it lets us see just how much stronger we can get!

To work out your FFMI, all you need to do is use the following equation: FFMI = (LBM in kg) / (height in meters)^2

So convert your lean body mass to kilograms, then divided it by the square of your height in meters. Entering in your sample numbers, it would be FFMI=(72.01) / (1.73)^2 = (72.01) / (2.99) = 24.08.

The *maximum* it is generally agreed that you can score here is 25. Any higher than that and people will (perhaps rightly) suspect that you may be using steroids. This was the finding according to one study that surveyed a lot of natural athletes to see where they would peak. This is your 'genetic limit' and beyond that, you'll only really be able to add fat. It's not a 'perfect' score either though and some individuals genuinely have been able to break through and go even further beyond (*Dragon Ball Z* quote...) even without steroids. But as a rule: this is how far you can expect to go.

So if you have an FFMI of 24.08 and the maximum is 25, that means you have achieved 96.32% of your genetic potential. You can start to picture just how much bigger you could potentially get.

Know this though: the closer you start to get to your genetic limit, the harder it will become to add on more muscle. This is why experienced athletes can often be quite jealous of beginners who still experience 'noob gains'. But it's good news if you're currently very skinny, because it means you'll be able to start really piling on the pounds quickly with the right regimen.

Calculating Your AMR and BMR

With that out the way, we can finally work out your AMR and BMR. So what exactly are these numbers?

Well your BMR is your 'Basal Metabolic Rate'. This is just how much energy (in calories) your body needs in order to live. This is assuming you're not moving at all – just lying there. Your body will still need to use up energy simply to maintain your systems – to help you blink, breathe, digest and pump blood around your body.

Your AMR is this number + the number of calories you are burning through movement and exercise. When you combine those two things, what you're left with is the total energy demand of your body on an average day. This in turn tells you just how much you need to eat if you want to avoid burning fat and how much you need to eat if you want to *encourage* burning fat.

Because if you were trying to lose weight, then you would need to remain in a *calorie deficit*. That would mean you'd be eating fewer calories than you burn throughout the day.

As a result, your body would be forced to burn fat in order to fuel your various movements or just to keep your heart beating.

But you're not trying to lose weight, in fact, you're trying to *gain* weight (albeit a certain kind). That means you need to maintain a caloric *surplus* where you consume more calories in the day than you use up. This in turn will mean that your body then has extra calories to spare and it will most likely store these calories as fat around the body. Or use them to build muscle. Or provide you with fuel to move around with.

You don't want to go *too* far into surplus or you'll end up looking huge and blobby while also breaking out in bouts of acne. Instead, you need to go just far *enough* into a surplus and that's why you need to get scientific and you need to calculate precisely how many calories you need and how many you're eating.

There are numerous equations for calculating BMR but the one we're going to use is based on your lean body mass. That's very important because muscle is more metabolically active than fat. If you are very heavy due to lots of muscle, then you will burn more calories simply to maintain and operate all that muscle mass!

So the equation looks like this: BMR = 370 + (9.79757519 x LBM(lbs))

When I take my 158.76 and put that in, I get a BMR of 1,925. That means that if I just lay there all day, I would lose weight unless I ate at least 1,925 calories (kcal).

Now let's add in activity. This is going to be something of a rough estimate but the following list should help:

- 1.2 if you're sedentary (little or no exercise)

- 1.375 if you're lightly active (you exercise 1-3 times a week)

- 1.55 if you're moderately active (you exercise or work about average)

- 1.725 if you're very active (you train hard for 6-7 days a week, or you do a job that requires a lot of time on your feet)

- 1.9 if you're highly active (you're a physical laborer or a professional athlete)

If you feel you're 'somewhere in the middle', then guestimate a number that's somewhere in the middle. Unfortunately, there's never a way to be *absolutely* sure.

Let's say you are around a 1.55 as you train a lot but you certainly are not near being a professional athlete or physical laborer. So that gives you an AMR of 2,983 which is actually quite average for a male (the average is generally thought to be about 2,500).

Using Fitness Trackers

Note that there are other ways you can calculate your calorie expenditure too. One example is simply to wear a good fitness tracker that includes a heart rate monitor. Some good examples include the Fitbit Surge, the Charge HR, the Microsoft Band 2 or Garmin Vivoactive HR. If you're reading this a few years in the future, then probably there are better models out there by now.

Either way, a fitness tracker works by using an optical sensor on the wrist to measure your heartrate throughout the day. The best models will take regular readings and combine this with information you entered about yourself and movement data picked up from a pedometer, gyroscope and accelerometer.

When all this information is collated, you can then be given a rough calorie burn estimate for any given day.

The other great thing is that you can sync this with My Fitness Pal, which is a smartphone app and website where you can log everything you eat. This lets you see your total calories in and out and will adjust the number whenever you go on a long walk, do a workout or perhaps have a day where you move very little.

And by comparing these two numbers you can make sure you stay in that surplus. If it's 11pm and you've been too active and haven't eaten much, you know you need to get busy and down some bulking powder!

Chapter 2 – Maintaining Your Caloric Surplus

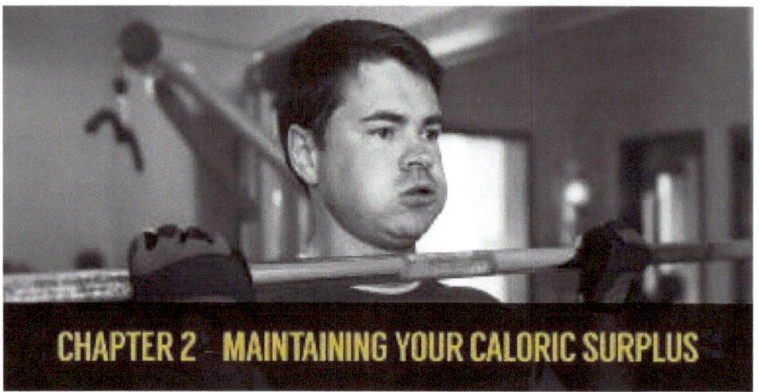

CHAPTER 2 - MAINTAINING YOUR CALORIC SURPLUS

So we've gone through all that just to get your calorie burn for the day. But this is absolutely crucial because maintaining a calorie surplus is going to be the *single most important factor* when it comes to bulking. As long as you are eating more than you are burning, then you *will* get bigger over time.

Why Your Calorie Surplus is So Important

So just why is a calorie surplus so important?

Well the first and most obvious reason is that building muscle *requires* energy. You're asking your body to construct new tissue from the protein in your diet and that means you're going to need to eat more to provide that energy.

The other reason is that you're trying to prevent the breakdown of muscle. When you're low on energy and your body is forced to burn fat, it goes into a catabolic state. First, your body notices that your stomach is empty. This causes a release of ghrelin the hunger hormone.

That then triggers the release of cortisol, the stress hormone, which is designed to encourage your brain to go and seek out food. Your body is now in a 'catabolic state' where it will burn fat and use it for fuel.

But that cortisol also triggers the release of something else: myostatin. Myostatin is one of the single biggest enemies of bodybuilders because it tells the body to breakdown muscle. Muscle is very energy demanding and *not* very energy efficient. As we've seen, simply having muscle increases your BMR.

Thus, if you are starving and your body is low on the sugars and ATP it needs to run, it's going to want to break down that muscle and certainly not prioritize it for building. What's more, is that this will release some additional energy that your body can then use.

So being in a calorie deficit puts you in an anxious, skinny, lean and efficient mode. Conversely though, when you eat large amounts of calories, it lets your muscles swell up because you're creating the right environment. Your body will store some of that 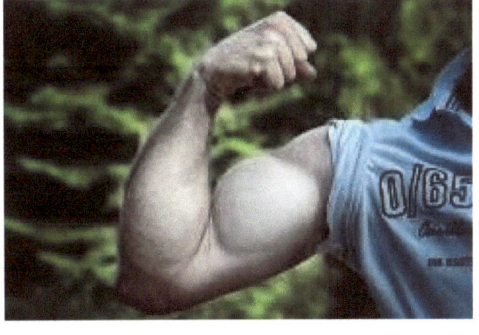 energy as glycogen, right in the muscle cells, to make them look even bigger. And when you provide the correct stimulus for growth, your system will respond by *building*.

This is also why rest is so important and why you need to train without exhausting yourself. The goal of training is not to burn calories, just to provide stimulus for growth.

You're aiming to get pumped in the gym and then spend the rest of the time eating and resting. I call this *living like a lion.*

How Many Calories Do You Need?

So the next question is just how many calories you actually need in order to bulk. Obviously this is dependent on the AMR as we just worked out… but how many *more* calories than that should you aim for?

The answer again varies and is dependent on various factors – such as whether you're more interested in a lean bulk (meaning you add muscle with very little body fat) or a 'dirty bulk' (meaning that you add both muscle *and* fat).

A very clean bulk is achievable with something like an additional 150-200 calories a day. A slightly clean bulk is around 200-300. And if you want to dirty bulk, you could go up to 400-450. Higher than that though and you're starting to get into fat territory, place a bit of a strain on your body and potentially case acne and other problems. This can also be unhealthy.

Which should you choose?

Well, if you're someone who is very skinny and you're just starting out then you can go for a pretty dirty bulk with a surplus of 300-400 calories. Because right now, you're probably in a position where you want to be a lot stronger. You may have tried to bulk in the past and been disappointed. But at the same time, you're a *noob* which means you have the potential for noob gains.

In other words, you have the potential to bulk up and *fast* if that's what you want to do. And in your current situation, it probably *is* what you want to do as well! What you can then do is to later do a short cutting cycle in order to bring your body fat back down and reveal the definition and striations.

Conversely, if you're someone who is an average size right now – perhaps a mesomorph – then you may well be a little stocky but also carrying a bit more fat than you want. If you're *already* at around 12-15% body fat, then you'll probably want to avoid adding too much extra and so in that case you'll do better to bulk a little slower without so much excess.

And finally, if you're someone who is at or around their genetic potential, or you're someone who is already in good shape, then a clean bulk is the safest way to go.

Chapter 3 – Understanding Macros

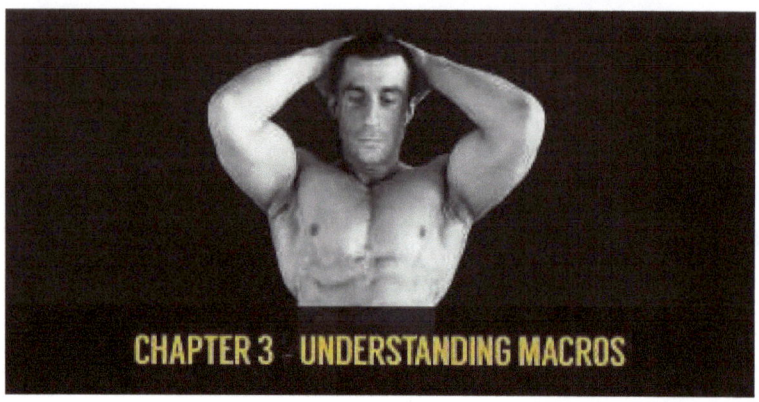

In bodybuilding circles, there is a diet called IIFYM. This stands for 'If It Fits Your Macros' and it essentially means that you can eat anything you like, as long as you eat within certain parameters. The concept began life on forums like Bodybuilding.com in fact as a response to a lot of inane questions. People were repeatedly asking: "Can I eat donuts?" or "Can I eat chicken with the skin on?" and the answer would always be: "Yes, if it fits in your macros!". This was eventually shortened to IIFYM (as a joke as much as anything) which eventually evolved to become practically a diet in and of itself. The IIFYM diet!

This is broadly speaking the diet that we're going to be following in order to bulk! However, there are certain caveats here as we're also going to see.

So perhaps the best place to start is: what is a macro?

Essentially, a macro is a 'macronutrient', which is effectively another term for a food group. Macronutrients include protein, carbohydrates and fats and together, these effectively make up your caloric intake. We don't count fiber because fiber doesn't contain any calories (it just passes straight through!).

Protein and carbs both count for 4 calories per gram. So if you eat 10 grams of protein, that is 40 calories. Fat meanwhile contains 9 calories per gram.

Seeing as you know that you can eat, let's say, 2700 calories, this then means you want to work backwards in order to decide how much of that is going to consist of protein, carbs and fats respectively. And the answer to this is going to depend once again on various different aspects regarding your biology.

Let's take a look...

Protein

When it comes to building muscle, the most important thing is

that you are eating a LOT of protein. Protein is basically meat and plant matter – carbon – and this is broken down to create amino acids. You may have heard that we are 'carbon based lifeforms' which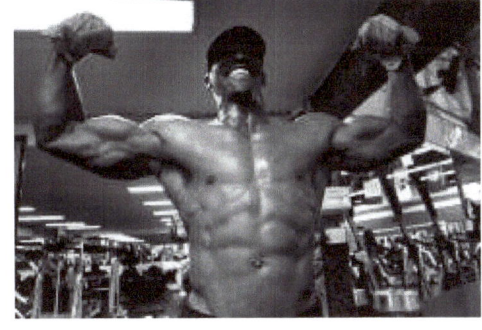

basically tells you that humans are *made* from carbon.

So when you consume protein, you are eating the literal building blocks that compose your body. This means protein can help you to repair cuts and bruises, to rejuvenate skin cells, to grow and crucially to grow *muscle*.

Thus begins the cycle of muscle building: you work out to break down your muscle fiber and then you provide your body with rest and with protein which allows it to restore it again and build it back up. If you're not getting the protein, then you're not providing your body with what it needs to restore muscle. And that means that you won't grow – in fact you'll just become weaker!

So now the question becomes how much protein you need. And fortunately, you have a very easy and simple answer for that question: 1 gram of protein for every lb of bodyweight. So if you weigh 170lbs, you need to eat 170 grams of protein. This will net you 680 calories, which means you now have 2,020 calories left to divide between fats and carbohydrates!

Why 1 gram for each pound? That's simply what has been shown to be optimal in studies. Countless studies have looked at this question and all of them have found that this amount leads to the optimal amount of muscle growth. And you can of course go above this number – heading closer to 1.2 or 1.3 grams (around 884 calories) but this will start to reach the point of 'diminishing returns'.

Energy

So now the question is where you'll get your energy from and the answer is that it again partly depends on you and on your aims.

Of course the objective is always going to be minimizing fat gain while maximizing muscle gain and in that regard there are two schools of thought.

One is that you should eat more carbs and less saturated fat.

And one is that you should eat more saturated fat and fewer carbs.

Tricky!

So perhaps it's best if we assess each stance. Those who favor saturated fat do so because they believe it will minimize weight gain. It can do this because saturated fat is a slow release form of energy. That is to say, that it takes a long time for the body to break it down and use it as energy. This means that it will slowly release energy into your bloodstream, thereby enabling you to go for longer without snacking *and* prevent you from getting a sudden sugar spike. The concern with carbs is that they quickly release their energy into the body, causing a sudden spike in blood sugar which is then immediately followed by a spike in insulin. That insulin causes the body to use up all of the available glucose in the blood, thereby leaving you feeling exhausted and drained. This is one reason that we often feel sleepy after we've eaten!

Saturated fat also has a lot of health benefits (the good kind), because it aids with nutrient absorption (helping you to get the goodness from your foods) and it encourages the production of testosterone (because testosterone is made from cholesterol). It's good for the brain and in general, it's a mistake to leave it out of the diet. Carbs on the other hand – specifically simple white carbs – tend to be processed, man-made food with lots of sugar.

These are 'empty calories' that don't provide any nutritional value and thus they aren't terribly good for the body.

But on the other hand, a lot of bodybuilders prefer to choose carbs as the dominant macro in their diet. This is because carbs are the body's preferred energy source. That means that if you eat lots of carbs, they're *more likely* to be used for energy during workouts and movements rather than being stored as fat. They also contain fewer calories in total, meaning that you can eat more of them without gaining lots of weight.

Some people go as far as to believe that they can effectively eat large amounts of carbs without really gaining too much excess body fat (see Vitruvian Physique's YouTube video on the subject). And there's more here too because carbs are actually the preferred energy source of fast twitch muscle fiber. Fast twitch muscle fiber (as opposed to slow twitch, the other type) is the type of muscle fiber that is used for powerful, explosive movements such as sprinting or lifting very heavy weights. As it happens, fast twitch muscle fiber is also *thicker* than slow twitch, meaning that a muscle composed of more fast twitch will be bigger.

On the other hand, the body prefers triglycerides (fats) when it comes to exercise that requires you to exert yourself over a long duration. This is true for jogging for example and for walking long distances. And that's the reason that running is so *great* for burning lots of fat and getting slimmer. You want fast twitch muscle fiber, so it makes sense to fuel it with carbs.

Note that not *all* carbs release sugar quickly. 'Slow carbs' or 'complex carbs' release energy much more slowly.

These are carbs that also contain a lot of fiber and/or fat and good examples include green vegetables, new potatoes, whole wheat bread, brown pasta, etc.

It's also important to note that not all carbs are empty calories. In fact, some carbs are *highly* nutrient dense and a good example of this is fruit! Fruit is a carb and it happens to be a fantastic source of vitamins, minerals and more. These have a ton of great health benefits which can help with bulking and are just generally very desirable – they can boost testosterone, prevent muscle breakdown, give you more energy, help you to sleep better and more.

So if both arguments are so compelling, what should you do? The answer is a) to find out what works best for you and b) find some kind of compromise. Personally, I split my macros roughly evenly between carbs and fats.

Chapter 4 – On Nutrients and Hormones

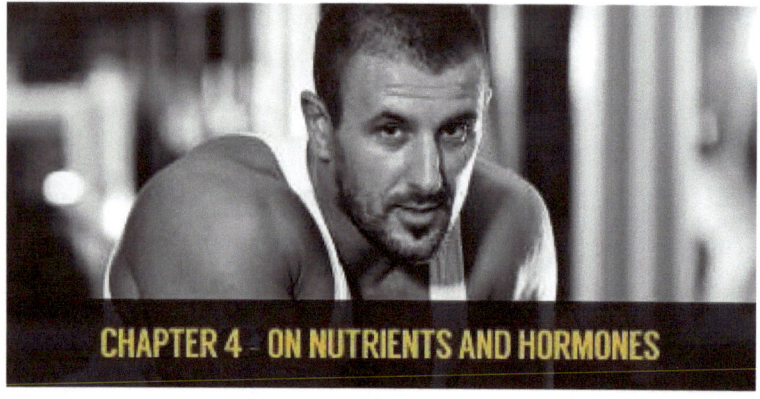

CHAPTER 4 - ON NUTRIENTS AND HORMONES

So now you can see how IIFYM works. Can you eat donuts and still build lean muscle? You sure can: as long as it fits your macros.

But there's a problem here and that problem is that it can lead to people eating some *seriously* unhealthy diets.

"I can eat donuts and still get into great shape? Great, then that's ALL I'm going to eat!"

The only problem with this strategy is that you're *only* consuming simple sugars and you're *only* consuming processed, man-made food. This then means that you won't be getting any vitamin C, D, A, B, E… and you won't be getting any omega 3 fatty acid, any CoQ10, any magnesium, potassium, calcium, zinc, iron… you get the picture!

All of these things have important and crucial roles in the body and can help us to improve the look of our skin, the strength of our bones, our brain power, our immune system, our hormones and much, much more.

Think of the people you know who eat nothing but junk food. They're probably either badly overweight, or spotty with bad hair and nails. This is not conducive to building muscle!

And thus, what's also highly important is to get your *micronutrients*. And that means that you need to be eating fruits, vegetables, fish, nuts and more. This is what will allow your body to operate optimally and in turn, it's what will ensure that you can build as much muscle as possible and also maintain the best possible health.

An easy rule for this is to try and go 'paleo'. Paleo is another popular diet which involves eating only foods that would have grown naturally. These are the foods our bodies evolved to thrive on and they include tons of nutrients. So the simple rule is that if 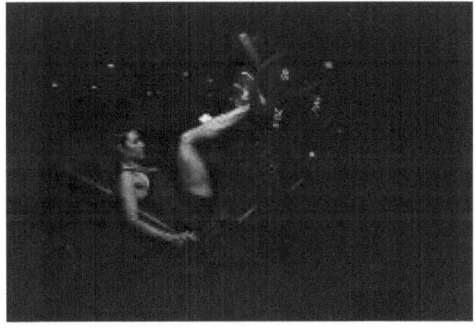 you couldn't hunt or forage it, you can't eat it!

Paleo is quite a strict diet though and especially if you combine it with IIFYM (just try ordering anything in a restaurant). And if you're trying to get lots of calories from carbs, it does help to be able to eat bread, pasta and rice.

So instead my version of this diet is the 'agricultural diet'. You can eat anything that would be in a paleo diet plus anything that could be grown or made on a farm. And of course I'm fairly relaxed with that: because I do sometimes fancy an ice cream or some chocolate and my macros allow for that... so why not? It's not that you *can't* eat processed foods – it's that you *must* eat the other stuff. And when you do, you will feel and perform much better, leading to better muscle mass.

So just be aware of this difference. Seek out complex carbs rather than simple carbs, eat lots of fruit and veg and keep the processed foods and empty calories to a minimum and make them treats!

Why Aren't I Growing? The Hormones Element

We haven't gotten to the exercise you need to do yet but that's because we've put things here in order of importance. Bulking is done predominantly in the kitchen, with the gym being the afterthought – not the other way around. *As long* as you are eating a calorie surplus and getting your grams of protein, then you will find that you are able to grow and bulk up and even add some muscle.

But some of you have probably tried 'eating a lot' in the past and found it didn't work. So the question now becomes why not?

If you've calculated your AMR, your macros and your regular calorie intake and you are maintaining a surplus... how can you not be growing?

You can ask this question on a forum and depending on where you ask, they'll tell you you're wrong! "It's simple math!" they say.

"If you eat more calories than you burn, it has to go somewhere and you will grow!" they say. "If you're not growing, you can't be eating enough calories. Are you skipping meals?"

But what they fail to consider is individual differences and just how much your AMR can vary depending on your hormonal makeup and other factors. You can run the numbers all you want and wear fitness trackers but there's certain things that they just can't tell you.

This is something that a lot of people deny who swear by calorie counting and IIFYM. They snort in derision at people who say that eating a low carb diet is useful as a way to manage insulin for example. But if you need proof that this *does* play a role, then you just have to look at someone who uses steroids.

Someone who uses steroids will build much more muscle and burn much more fat while doing the exact same routine as someone who *doesn't* use them (although they'd also suffer lots of side effects...). However, if they were to put their numbers in as we had done earlier, their AMR would be the exact same.

Steroids work by increasing testosterone (by binding to the androgen receptors). Now imagine what happens if you have *low* testosterone. And as it happens, a lot of guys *do* have low testosterone – which leads to them being weak, flabby and overweight.

Conversely, you might struggle to gain weight if you have a condition like hyperthyroidism. This is a genetic disorder that causes your metabolism to be very fast. It makes you anxious, jittery and thin and it's all to do with your balance of T3 and T4 hormones.

It's also possible to have hypothyroidism (note the 'o') which has the opposite effect and makes you tired, lethargic and overweight (while also causing problems like acne). In women, hypothyroidism can be the result of polycystic ovaries.

What's my point? Simply that you might be trying to bulk and not understanding why it's not working – only to eventually be diagnosed with hypothyroidism or hyperthyroidism! And in that case, you wouldn't be able to change size and shape but you also wouldn't know *why* you had that problem! Likewise, you could have low testosterone but not realize it and carry on in vain trying to gain more muscle mass.

But even if you don't have either of these conditions, there's a good chance that you could have *some* kind of imbalance or deficit that leads to similar problems. It's actually a mistake to think of your body *too* much in terms of being 'ill' or 'well'. In reality, our systems are not binary but they are spectrums. You don't have 'low testosterone' or 'high testosterone': you have a number somewhere between those two extremes. What's more, is that your testosterone levels are *constantly* fluctuating throughout the day – after you exercise, after you eat, while you sleep, when you're stressed, during sex. And they fluctuate more or less for different people. The same goes for insulin, myostatin, cortisol, T4...

So you might not have hyperthyroidism but you might be 'borderline'. You could have a very high metabolism that still falls *within* the normal range. No one is going to prescribe you any medication and yet your attempts to bulk will likely be met with failure.

So what do you do? The best strategy you have is to try and *change* your hormonal makeup for the better, while at the same time carefully monitoring your results and adjusting your approach.

Not gaining any weight with that 300 calorie surplus? Then you probably have a very fast metabolism that you're not picking up on, meaning that your surplus probably *isn't* really a surplus. Try increasing that number!

Meanwhile, you can slow down your metabolism with the way you eat. Continuously supplying yourself with complex carbs will do that, as will your training if you keep it up. The rest of the time, it can help to try and minimize stress which contributes to a faster metabolism by raising cortisol, adrenaline and noradrenaline.

And believe it or not – running long distance or going on long walks can also help! Why? Because this will help you to develop more cardio strength. In doing that, you can lower your resting heartrate, which will actually send signals to your brain that make you feel calmer. When you do this, you can then keep your cortisol lower throughout the day.

Likewise, if you're someone who struggles to lose weight, then you should try going low carb. This will force your body to learn to prefer fats as an energy source which in turn will help with your weight loss. It will also avoid those insulin spikes that make you hungry *and* lead to more fat storage. At the same time, try doing HIIT which uses up all of the sugar in the blood stream and muscles through intense bursts of energy and then forces you to turn to your fat stores.

Another thing to think about is the peaks and troughs in your metabolism and when the best *time* to eat is. If you want your carbs to go to your muscle, then you need to consume them when your glycogen stores are lowest – right after you've trained (that's called carb backloading). Likewise, if you want to build muscle overnight, then consuming a slow release form of protein (such as casein) is a good idea because it will help you to have all the protein you need just when you're in the deepest levels of sleep. Around 4am is the time when the body maximizes its production of testosterone and of growth hormone – which are the anabolic hormones that tell the body to build muscle. In the morning when you wake up, your blood sugar is low because you've gone all night without eating. This is great for losing weight but terrible for building muscle, so if you want to avoid it being a negative thing then you need to get some calories in you *early* to get out of that highly catabolic state.

As you can see then, you shouldn't think only in the short term and ask yourself how to quickly add lots of calories to your diet – you should also think in the long term and think about how what you're eating will change your body and help you to build more muscle over time by slowing down your metabolism.

But the simplest way to *start* bulking for most people is going to be to maintain a surplus. For *most* people that is more than sufficient and the AMR will be accurate. It's only when this fails that you then need to think about ways that you can slow your metabolism down *and/or* increase your surplus further. And you need to monitor your results as you do that to see what's working – so keep those scales out!

Chapter 5 – IIFYM IRL

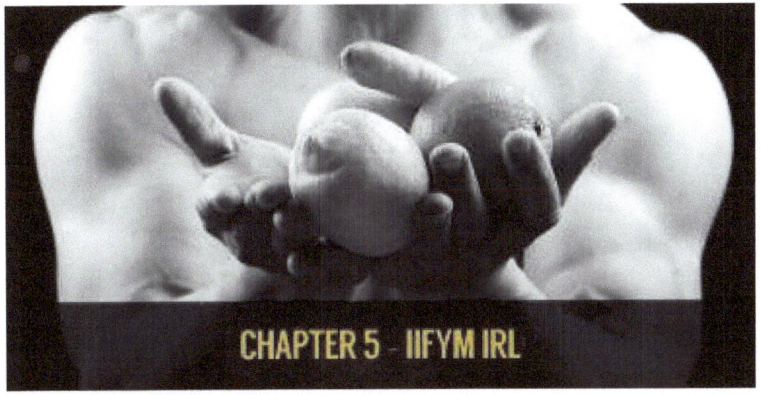

CHAPTER 5 - IIFYM IRL

Sorry, I just couldn't resist the temptation to use two acronyms like that right next to each other. Of course IRL stands for 'In Real Life' and what I'm talking about here is how you're going to get all these concepts to work in the real world. How can you take that concept and make it work as a part of your routine?

It's all very well and good telling you to eat all these calories and to eat loads of protein... but where can you find those things? How can you afford it? And how to you force it all down without wanting to throw up?

In other words, you need to find ways to make this actually *practical* so that it will work with your routine. And to do that, you need to get strategic.

This is incredibly important and it's the thing that people all-too-often forget. If you're trying to bulk up, then you need to find a way to stick to your training and your diet. That means it needs to be *realistic*. It's better to have very modest aims and actually stick to them, than it is to be incredibly ambitious and end up not doing any of the things you set out to do!

So let's consider some tips that will help you out...

What to Eat

The majority of your results will come from your diet. Supplements are just that – *supplements*. They should be supplemental to a good diet and never viewed as a *substitute* for one.

So then the question is, what kinds of foods can you eat that will satisfy all the criteria we've been looking at in the chapters so far? What will help you keep your protein and calories high, while also being nutritionally dense and slow release? What leaner sources of protein are there for when you're trying to lean bulk?

Here are some foods that will help you a great deal...

Tuna – Tuna is one of the THE most convenient options when it comes to finding lean sources of protein. Canned tuna is *very* affordable while containing 20 grams or more of protein in many cases. It's lean, it's versatile and it's tasty too. PLUS it's also good for the brain thanks to that omega 3 fatty acid content. The only downside? Consuming too much can risk a potential mercury overdose... not good!

Salmon – Salmon is not quite as low in calories as tuna (a good thing for bulking!) but it's just as high in protein and omega 3 fatty acid. The better news? It doesn't have the mercury problem. The downside? It's much more expensive...

Avocado – These are all the rage among the low-carb crowd at the moment, which is owing to their delicious taste, their healthy fats and their large range of other health benefits.

They're quite calorific but healthy at the same time, so they make a great way to add more calories and fat to pretty much any meal!

Oil – Adding sunflower or vegetable oil to your food isn't actually bad for you! But it *does* contain a LOT of calories, which is another really good way to sneak them in when you're starting to feel full and struggle to keep eating more...

Eggs – Eggs are high in protein as well as the healthy saturated fats AND choline (great for the brain). The best part about eggs though is that they are a 'complete protein'. This means that they contain *all* of the essential amino acids that the human body needs to 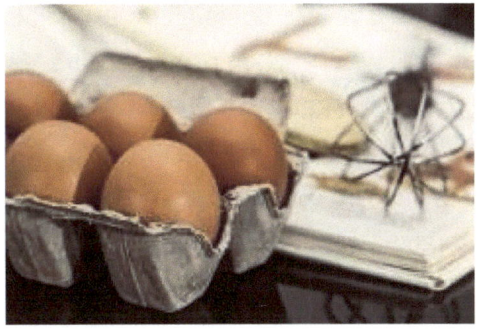 function. There are very few complete protein sources in the world, so this makes egg pretty special.

Sweet Potatoes – A good source of carbs that's also nutritious and high in slow-release complex carbs.

Chicken – Chicken is another very lean protein source and this time it doesn't come with any significant downsides. You can eat chickens until the cows come home.

Beef – And cows until the chickens come home? Beef is also an excellent source of protein, which is partly due to some very interesting additional nutrients it contains. Specifically, beef is actually one of the only natural sources of CoEnzyme Q10 and of creatine – both of which give you more energy and drive during your workouts!

Rice – If you're looking for a carb that is fairly easy to eat in bulk, then rice is a good bet!

Nuts – Nuts are also great. Not only do these provide fiber but they're also a very good source of protein, calories and good fats. They also provide various micronutrients like zinc, selenium and magnesium.

Milk – Milk is one of the very best things you can keep around the house if you're bulking and especially full fat milk. Remember: milk is where whey protein *comes from* and when you drink milk, you're still getting a lot of that whey in there. In fact, a glass of milk contains 3.4grams of protein, while full fat milk is widely considered one of the very best things you can drink if you want to give yourself more healthy fats.

Butter – A good butter is another very useful tool for packing on more calories. Wish your food was a little more calorific? Then just butter it up! You can even try the 'Bulletproof Coffee' that everyone is talking about by dropping a stick of butter in your morning brew!

Oats – Oats are great at adding more stodge and at giving you more slow-release energy. Add these to a shake and they'll increase the calories while also helping you to have more energy for work, play and workouts!

Bulk Eating Tips

Try GOMAD

Have you tried absolutely everything to bulk up with no success? Not sure where to turn? It's enough to make you go mad… or at least GOMAD! GOMAD stands for 'Gallon Of Milk A Day' and is considered a last chance saloon when all else has failed. As the name rather implies, this is a method of eating that has just ONE simple rule: you have to drink a whole gallon of milk every single day.

When you do this, you'll find that it's enough to help you pack on muscle thanks to the huge amounts of protein, calories AND saturated fat. It can greatly increase your testosterone and your growth hormone among other things and some reports suggest that it's *nearly* as effective as a steroid cycle if you're new!

Of course it also carries some health risks and it's not a good idea to consume *anything* in massive quantities normally. So if you're going to try this method, the key is to get in and out *quickly*.

Find a Salad Bar

One of the best things you can possibly do to improve your chances of bulking success is simply to find a convenient place where you can get lots of calories without spending too much or breaking from your usual routine. A salad bar is a great place to find this as they tend to be all you can eat while also serving up eggs, pasta and other good stuff for your bulking goals. They tend to be pretty cheap as well!

Stay Consistent

One of the single most useful things you can do to make tracking your calorie intake that bit easier is just to stay consistent. In other words, have a few meals that you eat regularly and that way you'll know exactly the calories and macros you're getting without having to do the math every time or input them anew. It might not be terribly exciting but this is a big help.

Use MyFitnessPal

You can of course log all of your calories in a diary or notebook but this is a lot of work and takes a lot of time. Instead then, consider logging your calories using the excellent app, 'MyFitnessPal'. This will allow you to simply scan anything you eat to get its barcode and that will then automatically fill in all the details for you!

Chapter 6 – Adding Supplements

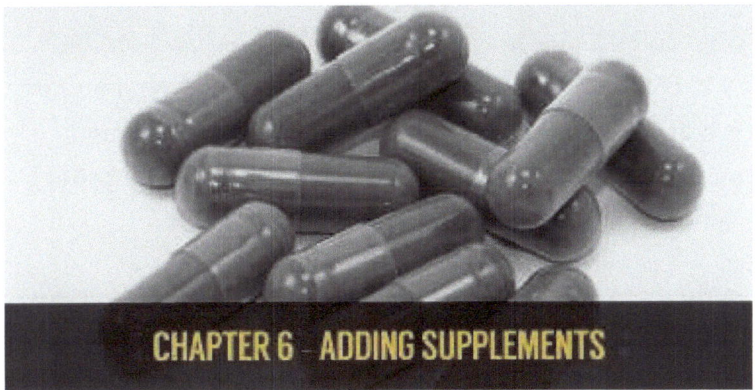

CHAPTER 6 - ADDING SUPPLEMENTS

Supplements can greatly help in your bid to build muscle and size and they're a great way to get your protein, nutrients and more. Your diet is still number one but it definitely doesn't hurt to add a few of the right supplements too. And this would hardly be a complete bulking book without at least touching on a few...

Of course the big one here is going to be protein shake. The most popular form of protein shake is called whey protein and this is a by-product of the cheese making process that comes from milk. It's a lean source of protein and it also has good 'bioavailability' (basically meaning your body can use it).

When you buy whey protein it will come in the form of a shake that you can easily mix with water. This is a tasty treat, it's actually very affordable and you can drink it anywhere you are. It's lean too (so ideal for those who are trying a lean bulk) and it doesn't cost that much compared with eating lots of meat.

What all this means is that whey protein provides one of the most convenient methods available for getting the amount of protein you need in order to bulk.

A single shake can get you anything from 20 to 50 grams of protein and you can have two or three a day. But for those who just want to bulk and aren't bothered by how *clean* the bulk is, then you can go one step further and use a weight gainer instead. This is a protein shake *plus* a huge amount of calories and carbohydrates to fuel you with energy and often with other supplements (like BCAAs, creatine, etc.) as well.

Do you *need* to take a protein shake or weight gainer? Certainly not. In fact, you don't *need* any supplements at all!

But what you'll find is that it can be a real struggle to reach your calorie and protein goals otherwise. When combined with the right diet and the right training, this can be enough to really accelerate your growth and help you to get much bigger, much faster. And if you're new to all this, then why not set yourself up for a win?

Of course there are other supplements you can use for bulking too – though none quite so useful or game-changing as the shakes.

One example of something worth checking out, is creatine. Creatine is a supplement that is very popular among Olympic athletes and others, thanks to its ability to improve cellular energy. It does this by recycling the ATP used by the muscles (ATP being the purest source of energy) allowing for a few extra seconds of maximum exertion. This can be pretty helpful in the gym when you're going all out but that's *not* actually why we're interested in it!

Instead, we're interested in creatine because it also happens to have the ability to increase fluid retention in the muscles. When you consume creatine, it encourages the muscles to store more glycogen and water which in turn makes them actually appear slightly larger. That's right: just by using creatine you can actually see your muscles increase in size by about an inch!

Then there are the other supplements. You have things like your BCAAs, which can help to prevent the breakdown of muscle, you have things like testosterone boosters (one example being tribulus terrestris) and then you have your pre-workouts. While these can all help to some small degree, they're also expensive and quite complicated. The small amount of benefit they provide – as a general rule – won't be worth the time or the expense. And so for that reason, it makes a lot more sense to stick with protein shake/weight gainer and *perhaps* creatine. Don't bog yourself down with the rest unless you're starting to reach that 'genetic potential' level where you really do need every last bit of help you can get!

Oh, one more small thing I *would* recommend actually is to take some sort of multivitamin. We've already seen the importance of micronutrients: vitamin C prevents muscle breakdown (and may actually be one of the most overlooked contributing factors to muscle gain!); calcium helps to strengthen your bones, your connective tissues and your muscle contractions; vitamin D improves sleep and boosts testosterone production... the list goes on!

And apart from anything else, when you're working out that hard in the gym, it really does pay to give yourself all of the help you can get with regards to repairing your body and keeping your immune system strong. A vitamin supplement could be the difference between continuing your workout or having to take months off due to illness!

Chapter 7 – The Workouts

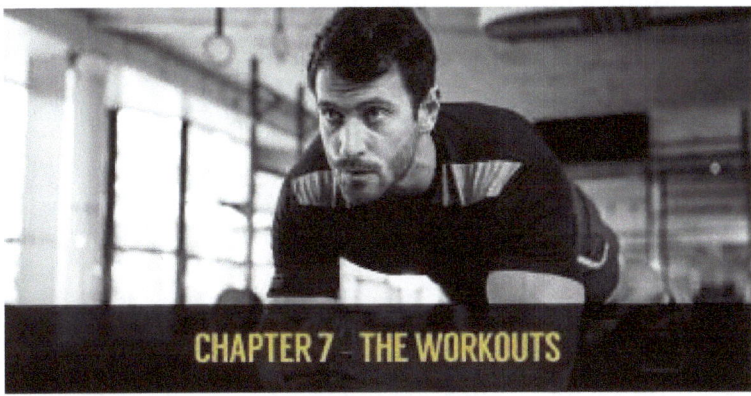

CHAPTER 7 - THE WORKOUTS

So far, this has been a book about eating. And so it should be! Eating is the *key* to bulking up.

But of course training had to come in somewhere sooner or later and unfortunately there's just no avoiding it! So how do you need to work out if you're planning on bulking?

How Training Builds Muscle

To answer this question, the first thing to consider is *how* exactly working out will add muscle in the first place. And the answer is that it can work through two separate mechanisms.

The first is that lifting weights creates microtears in your muscle fiber. In other words, the mechanical tension is great enough to cause tiny rips in your muscles that are too small to see or really feel

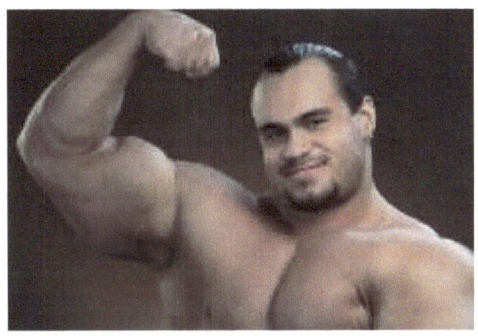

but which trigger the body to make repairs.

Then, when you rest later on, your system will use amino acids from your diet in order to restore those muscle fibers while also making them thicker and stronger in the process.

The other way it works is by increasing the glycogen stored in the muscle. When you lift weights, this causes a build-up of blood which makes them feel swollen – it's what you may know as 'the pump'. Along with the build-up of blood though are a number of metabolites such as testosterone and growth hormone. This then triggers more growth in the area too and leads to more glycogen being stored for better muscle endurance going forward.

In order to stimulate maximum growth in your muscles, you need to do *both* these things. But at the same time, you also need to avoid training too intensely for too long. This is a classic mistake: people who want to bulk up think they need to train more and train harder to do it! The problem is that when you train with great intensity for a long duration, you burn through a lot of calories and create a lot of stress (resulting in the release of stress hormones like cortisol). This combines to put the body into more of a catabolic state again and that thereby causes the breakdown of muscle – just like being hungry does!

So the key is to provide just enough microtears and just enough metabolites to trigger growth and then to rest for the remainder of the time! This is what author Tim Ferriss refers to as the MED or 'Minimum Effective Dose'.

And it's great news for you because it means you don't need to spend hours in the gym every day to get into shape – in fact you *mustn't*!

How to Lift for Size

So the question is how you go about lifting in such a way that you are going to create those necessary triggers for growth.

And the answer is that you should use isolation movements and drop sets. Not sure what they are? Read on!

Isolation

An isolation movement is any movement in the gym that involves lifting weights using only one joint. So an example of an isolation movement would be a bicep curl because only the elbow moves. On the other hand, the squat is a multi-joint exercise and so we call it a compound exercise.

Isolation movements are currently not in vogue with the hipster/paleo crowd but they remain the very best way to create tears and build up metabolites. That's because they let you focus on just one muscle until it is completely exhausted. Conversely, when you reach failure in the squats, it will likely be the combination of muscles that can no longer lift the weight – with no *one* muscle group being completely exhausted. Isolation movements also allow you to lift heavier and for longer, without risking injury.

(That said, compound movements have their benefits too – because they involve more muscles for example they increase the amount of metabolites you produce *on the whole*. For that reason, it doesn't hurt to start a workout with some squats or bench presses before moving on to your isolation work.)

Drop Sets

So once you're focussing on just one muscle group with a lat pull down, a bicep curl, a dumbbell row or a pec fly, you then need to make sure that you're creating both tears and the build-up of metabolites.

But there's a problem here. That's because creating microtears means you need to use a very heavy weight for a lower number of repetitions. You give up when you can't do any more reps and because the weight is so heavy, this will likely have caused some muscle damage in the process. But to build up metabolites, you need to 'occlude' the muscle. In other words, you need to redirect a lot of blood and nutrients to it where they'll pool and collect – and the best way to do this is with a slightly lighter weight curled for higher repetitions.

Try it: it's the former that gives you DOMS (Delayed Onset Muscle Soreness – the painful muscles you get the next day) and the latter that leads to the best pump *in* the gym.

And that's where the drop set comes in. This basically means you're going to train by starting out with very heavy weights and doing just a few repetitions. But then, when you reach failure and can't do any more, that's when you're going to drop those weights, move down the rack and pick up the next heaviest. You'll find that by dropping the weight slightly, you're now able to pump out a few more repetitions.

And then you drop down again.

And again.

And by the end, you'll be barely able to lift the lightest weight in the gym and your arms will feel crippled!

But this works like *magic*. That's because you're constantly challenging yourself and pushing through failure but also because you're managing to lift the heaviest weights possible while still doing a large volume of work. Remember: there's no pause in between the drops. Drop three or four times, then rest for one minute and then start again!

That said, this is just *one* intensity techniques and there are others too. These include things like doing pre-exhaust sets, or pyramid sets. Either way, the key is to try and feel the burn and the pump – if you don't get that feeling, then you aren't training hard enough.

Your Program

So that's how you lift the weights, now the question is which body parts to focus on and when. And for how long?

As a general rule, for bulking you shouldn't need more than 3 days of training a week and perhaps 4 at a push. This way, you'll have plenty of days to rest in between and you'll avoid burning too many calories or getting burned out and suffering with adrenal fatigue. The other good news is that each of those sessions need only last about 40 minutes.

And each of these 40 minute sessions can include a few different body parts. If you're using a drop set for instance, then three sets will be enough and you can then move on to another exercise for the same muscles. You might go from a bicep curl drop set, to performing some basic chin ups.

This will further breakdown the muscle but after you've completed this for about 3 exercises, you can then move onto the next body part. You will find you can fit two or three body parts into those 40 minute sessions then and here the key is to consider how well different muscle groups complement each other.

For example, if you're doing chest exercises, then it makes sense to do triceps and/or shoulders the same day. Why? Because a lot of exercises actually use these muscles in conjunction, meaning that going from bench press to shoulder press will somewhat pre-exhaust you for the latter.

The best way to formalize this is with PPL or 'Push, Pull, Legs'. Here, you simply spend one day of the week doing pushing exercises (bench press, shoulder press, press ups), one day with all the pulling exercises (pull ups, shrugs, bicep curls) and one day with the legs. This is a fantastic split for beginners because it allows you to intensely focus on each muscle group but not entirely for one session.

So 40 minutes of PPL, three times a week. That's your bulking prescription!

Chapter 8 – Closing Comments and Living the Lifestyle

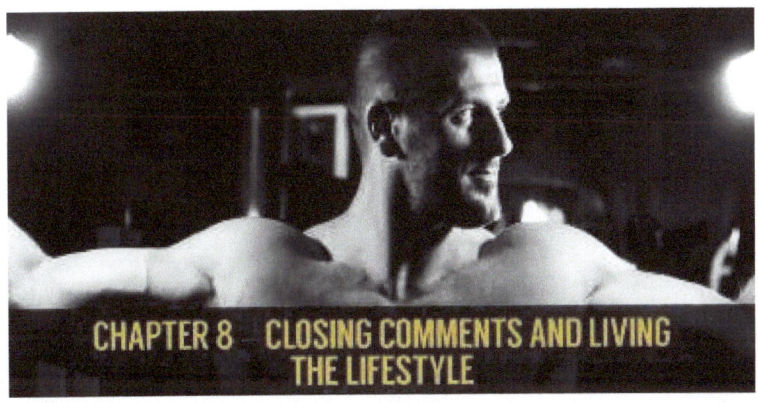

So if you combine that exercise with the diet we've recommended, then you'll find it's almost impossible *not* to grow. Of course you may need to tweak your precise calorie intake or macros as we mentioned before but for the vast majority of people, bulking can be as simple as doing PPL while getting some more protein and carbs.

And hopefully, you'll now know some ways you can do those things conveniently without too much disruption to your regular

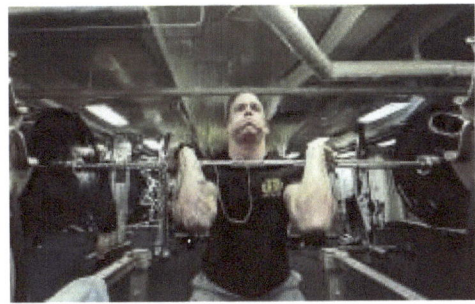

lifestyle. This is key because it means you actually stand a good chance of *sticking* at your new goals.

Finally, remember that your body is always going to be in one of two states: catabolic meaning you're anxious and burning muscle and fat, or anabolic meaning that you're growing.

We grow when we're well fuelled and we grow when we're rested.

So eat big, rest big and get BIG!

The body is changing all the time, it's simply a matter of us choosing whether we want it to change for the better or the worse...

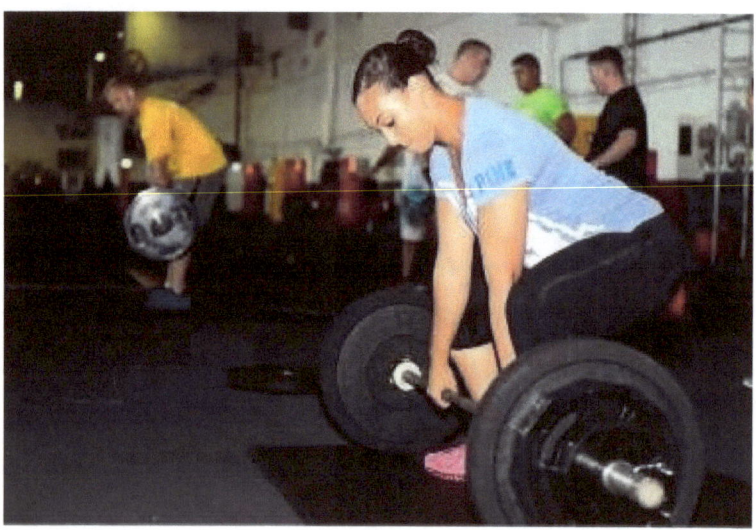

Cheat Sheet: Your PPL Workout Guide

The book went into how to eat for size in a lot of detail. Now it's time to think about the training. And what was the routine that we recommended? That was something called PPL.

This sheet is your cheat sheet to training – bring it with you to the gym and follow it to the letter. Over time, feel free to start swapping out exercises for new ones!

Primer: What is PPL?

PPL stands for 'Push, Pull, Legs'. This is a workout routine spread over three days, that challenges you to train your pushing muscles (pecs, triceps, shoulders), pulling muscles (biceps, lats) and legs (quads, hamstrings, calves) all on separate days.

You are to perform three workouts, ideally equally spaced through the week. Don't try to do more for the first 6 months at least.

This is enough to stimulate growth, while being sustainable and while avoiding injury or fatigue.

Train with intensity. That means you're not resting between sets and you're *always* training to failure or beyond.

But don't get out of breath! The aim is to breakdown muscle, this is *not* a fitness workout. Fitness workouts burn muscle! You can combine this with lots of walking in order to take care of your cardiovascular health.

Without further ado…

The Workout

<u>Push Day</u>

1 Bench Press – 1 x Warmup Set - 3 x 8 Reps to Failure

Start with the bench press. This is the big compound muscle for chest and you need to start with it before you fatigue other muscles and thereby lose the ability to exert maximum force.

Start with a warmup set. The best warmup for the gym is to practice the movements you're about to be doing but lighter. Then move on to the 'working sets'. You will be doing 3 x 8 repetitions, meaning the weight should be heavy enough that you could *not* do 9.

Chest Press – 2 x Drop Set

The chest press is a resistance machine and one that you can use to do isolation movements while also focussing very much on one body part without risk of dropping the weight.

The last set is a drop set. This means you're starting with a heavy weight (around your 3 rep max), then dropping it down each time you reach failure with no pause in between. This will allow you to go well beyond failure and really feel the microtears. Stop when the weight gets ridiculously light.

Pec Fly – 3 x 12 Reps to Failure

The pec fly is excellent for targeting the pecs and is especially useful because it allows you to apply stress in the stretched position.

Incline Dumbbell Press – 2 x 8 Reps

Now onto the incline bench press. This shifts the focus slightly onto the shoulders. We're doing it after a short gap, to give us time to recover from the bench press.

Lateral Raises, Upward Raises, Reverse Flyes – 2 x 12 Reps Each

Using light weights, you're going to perform a superset with these three exercises. This means you're performing them back to back, with no break in between. These moves target the three major 'muscle heads' of the shoulders, the side, front and rear delts.

Tricep Push Downs – 3 x 10 Reps

Tricep push downs are a great move for focusing on the triceps. They should already be sore from all the work they put in on the other movements here.

Dips – 2 x 12

End on dips, which will hit the pecs *and* the triceps in a big way.

<u>Pull Day</u>

Chin Ups – 3 x 10 Reps

Start with chin ups. These will hit the biceps with a relatively light exercise that's as compound as it gets for pulling motions.

Preacher Curls – 3 x 12 Reps to Failure, With Forced Reps

Preacher curls are curls performed on a bench to truly isolate the bicep muscles. These will cause maximum muscle damage.

Use forced reps by getting a friend to help you through the last few, or by using your other hand.

Hammer Curls – 3 x 8 Reps to Failure

Bicep curls with a neutral grip.

Pull Ups – 3 x 10 Reps

These are chin ups with an overhand grip, to target the lats more.

Lat Pull Downs – 3 x 10 Reps

Bent Over Rows – 3 x 10 Reps

Hanging Leg Raises – 3 x 10 Reps

Throwing some ab stuff in with the lats makes a lot of sense, seeing as hanging movements are ideal for working the upper abs.

Crunches – 2 x 20 Reps

<u>Leg Day</u>

This is the 'big compound lifts' day, that you will use to stimulate massive testosterone and growth hormone release.

Deadlift – 3 x 5 Reps

Stat with the deadlift and perform 3 x 5 reps. This trains almost the entire body!

Squat – 3 x 5 Reps

Moving straight into the equally difficult but more legs focussed squat. Don't go all the way to failure on either of these, for fear of injury.

Dumbbell Clean and Press – 3 x 10 Reps

This is a brutally exhausting move that involves picking dumbbells up off the floor and then pressing them overhead. This should just wake up those pulling and pushing muscles, while also once again being a truly 'full body' movement.

Calf Raises – 3 x 15 Reps

The calves are a seriously underappreciated muscle group, don't ignore them!

Leg Press – 3 x 12 Reps to Failure

Once again demonstrating the importance of resistance machines, the leg press will allow you to go right to failure with a legs move, with no risk of injuring yourself.

Leg Extensions – 3 x 12 Reps

Hamstring Curls – 3 x 12 Reps

Lunge Walking – 3 x 20 Steps

Finally, make a fool of yourself by walking around the room stepping into deep lunges while holding dumbbells on either side of you!

Your legs will be shaking like mad after this workout, so make sure to hold onto the handrails on the way out of the gym if it has stairs!

Resource Sheet: Build Your Home Gym

The easiest way to train if you're pushed for time, is to build your own gym!

This resource sheet will list all of the items you need to create a gym that you can use to train your entire body from home with ease!

Pull Up Bar

If you only get one item to train with from home, it should be a pull up bar. A pull up bar instantly gives you the ability to train your biceps and lats using your body weight – these are the only muscle groups that are normally a challenge when you have no equipment.

Best of all, a pull up bar will normally only set you back about $5. If you're struggling to find space in your home for one, then look into an 'iron gym' which will fit into your doorframe with no need to put holes in the frame.

Dumbbells

The next port of call is to get yourself a pair of dumbbells. Dumbbells will let you do even more training for your biceps and lats, this time using weights to provide much more resistance. The great thing about dumbbells though is that you can also use them to train just about every other body part – from your shoulders with shoulder presses to your pecs with dumbbell presses.

You can also do tricep kickbacks, upward rows and all manner of other things – and together, you should find that this allows for pretty much any type of workout that you can imagine.

In order to get the full benefit from this though, you'll need to find dumbbells with adjustable weights. In other words, you need weights that allows you to add and remove plates in order to increase and decrease the difficulty.

Again, dumbbells are quite cheap. Normally though, you'll buy them in a set that comes with about 20kg in weight. You'll want to build this up over time!

Weight Bench

A weight bench will be necessary if you want to start performing bench presses, dumbbell presses, bent over rows and all the rest from the comfort of your own home. Get an adjustable one and that way, you'll also have the option to do shoulder presses, incline and decline exercises.

Kettlebell

You aren't likely to be able to perform squats in your home unless you have an entire garage you can dedicate to training and use to store a whole squat rack and barbell in. Instead then, consider using a kettlebell instead. This is a large heavy ball with a handle attached that you can use to perform swings and even 'front squats' in order to train your legs at home.

Gymnastic Rings

Want to get creative? Gymnastic rings will let you perform ring dips, inverse push ups and even the iron cross from the comfort of your home! They're cheaper than TRX but do all of the same things. They hang neatly from your pull up bar to use and store easily when not needed!

Mindmap

The key to bulking is to train BIG, rest BIG, eat BIG
* Train just enough to stimulate growth
* Not enough to break down muscle
* Eat large amounts of protein and carbs
* Rest a lot
* Prioritize sleep
* Maintain a chilled outlook

Your goal is to:
* Maintain a calorie surplus
* Stay around 300 over your AMR
* Eat 1 gram of protein for 1lb of body weight
* Eat a nutrient dense diet

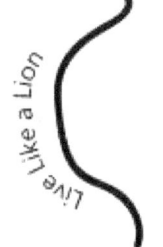

Live Like a Lion

Your Diet Goals

PPL is 'Push Pull Legs
Spend one day training
pushing muscles, pulling
muscles and legs respectively

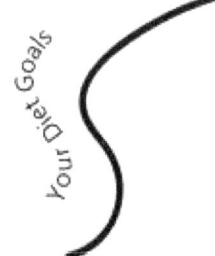

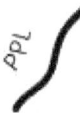

PPL

bulk like the hulk

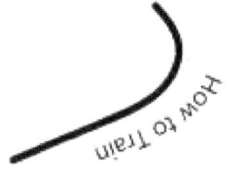

How to Train

Supplements

Top Tips for Getting Bigger Faster

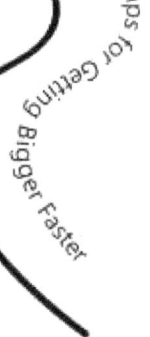

The aim is to break down muscle and to flood it with metabolites.

Train to and past failure. use longer sets of around 8-15.

Train to feel the 'pump' and the 'burn'.

Don't train too intensively or frequently, or you will burn muscle!

Supplements are optional but can help.
* Protein shake
* Creatine
* A multivitamin of some sort

* Make sure your new program isn't too ambitious
* Make sure it fits in your routine
* Manage your energy levels
* Make room in your life for training!

Other Fitness Books by This Author

If you would like to read more about Senior Health and Fitness, here is a list of the CreateSpace links, titles and descriptions:

https://www.createspace.com/6622994

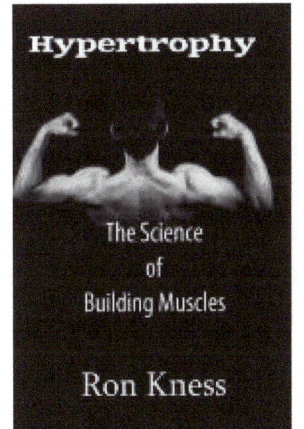

Hypertrophy – The Science of Building Muscles

Discover the secrets to muscle growth, supreme strength and maintaining a healthy diet!

So how on Earth are you going to magically build muscle?

Well, actually there is no magic. Unless you count powerful information as magic (and you should), there is no spells and magic potions here.

Instead, we are going to replace magic with a structured plan that if you follow, will lead to incredible results.

What you'll discover in this Book:

- The difference between fast and slow twitch muscle fiber

- The difference between 'sarcoplasmic' and 'myofibrillar' hypertrophy

- How to combine different types of training to experience 'athletic aesthetics'

- Why both compound AND isolation movements are perfectly valid

- How to train faster for better results

- How to use the Joe Weider intensity principles

- How to see growth even as a 'hard gainer'

- How to become incredibly lean and ripped, even as an endomorph - a person who has a hard time gaining weight

- How to work out your 'training philosophy'

- How to choose a fitness movement that works for you

- ...and much, much more!

This book will tell you everything you need to know to get into the gym tomorrow and start building a new body.

https://www.createspace.com/6114822

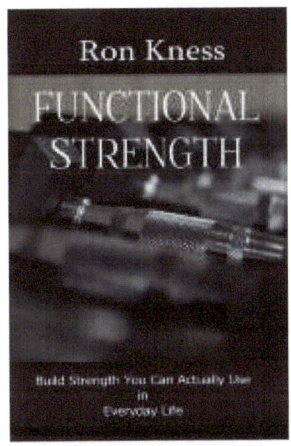

Functional Strength – Build Strength You Can Use In Everyday Life

Health and fitness fads come and go all the time but unfortunately not all of them are worth your time and effort. Some of them don't work, some of them are over-hyped and some of them are just plain dangerous.

But 'functional strength' is different. While functional strength is very much in vogue right now, it's not a 'fad' by any means. In fact, functional strength is the opposite of a fad and it's a step in the right direction for all of fitness.

That's because functional strength take it all back: takes it all back to the reasons that most of us started training in the first place. Or at least the reasons we should be training.

When you train for functional strength and fitness, everything becomes easier: from opening a jam jar, to helping a friend move furniture, to getting out of bed in the morning.

And if you want to train for your appearance as your first priority? Well then this is still the right way to go: because when you train for strength and power, you look much better. Don't believe me?

Then think about it logically: the reason that humans find healthy people attractive is because we assume they have better genetics and are better able to protect themselves and their families.

Someone with functional strength really can do all those things and really is healthier – so they send all of those unconscious signals that make them more attractive to the opposite sex!

Learn how to build strength that will not only improve everyday life, but also your appearance.

https://www.createspace.com/5520238

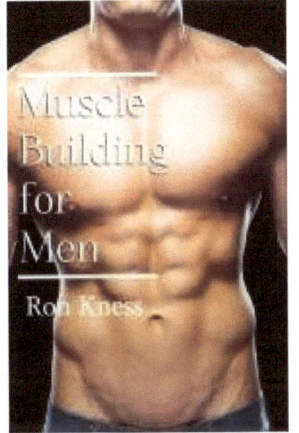

Muscle Building for Men - An Introductory Guide to Building Muscle Mass

In this book, I reveal a successful method of building muscle. Your best bet is to formulate an all-over workout routine that helps you do three things:
• Burn fat
• Build muscle mass
• Strengthen your muscle

Burn Fat

Burning off fat is really a quite simple process. All you have to do is burn more calories than you take in. In fact you have to burn 3,500 more calories per week than you take in to lose one pound of weight. One of the best ways to burn fat is through cardio-type exercises, such as running, biking or playing any sport that keeps you moving all the time and gets both your heart rate and breathing up into the fat burning zones – a target rate that is 80% of 220 minus your age.

Build Muscle Mass

While cardio burns off excess calories and the fat and weight associated with it, the only way to build muscle is through weight or strength training. Working with light weights but numerous repetitions will tone and tighten muscles for a well-defined look, but if you want to actually build muscle mass, you have to lift heavier weights, but fewer repetitions.

Strengthen your muscle

While getting leaner by burning off fat and building muscle mass are two ways to help strengthen your muscles, what we are talking about here is healthy eating. Without a proper diet, the other two will be harder to achieve. Part of losing weight and getting stronger is not only burning more calories, but taking in less calories to begin with.

What many people new to muscle building don't understand is that you actually are going to eat more food, but consume fewer calories. The key is to eat the right kinds of food; foods that will fuel your fat loss, build muscle and overall strengthen your muscles.

https://www.createspace.com/6668129

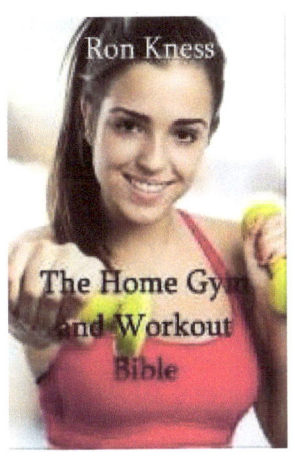

The Home Gym and Workout Bible

Discover How To Get In The Best Shape Of Your Life Without Ever Leaving The Comfort Of Your Home...

Although many people think going to a gym is the best way to get in shape, here's why you should consider working out from home...

- You don't have to "get up and go" to the gym or anywhere else... You just have to walk a few feet to your in-home gym

-It's easier to stay focused and avoid skipping days

- You can get started on a budget if you can't afford equipment (in many cases, working out at home will cost you less than a gym membership over time)

- You can get results faster because you're able to work on your fitness more often

- If you're overweight, starting at home makes it a lot easier to get going

Although there are a lot of advantages to working out from home, many people struggle with it. That's because, with a home workout program, the details are important...

When you do things the right way, you'll be burning fat and building muscle in just a few short weeks... you truly will get in the best shape of your life.

But, if you do things the wrong way, you could put yourself at risk of wasting your time, getting frustrated, spending money on equipment that you don't need, and ultimately even putting yourself at risk for injury.

To avoid all of that and get the best results with your home workout plan, you really an expert to help you get setup and make sure you do things the right way.

Because there's a lot of bad information about setting up a home gym online, I've put together a step-by-step guide to getting going the right way.

This is the next best thing to having a fitness expert in your home getting you setup and keeping you motivated...

Introducing "*The Home Gym and Workout Bible*". Get it now and start getting into the best shape of your life ... right from home!

About the Author

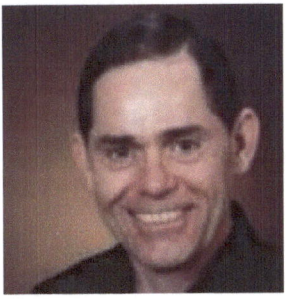

I grew up in Central Minnesota, where my parents owned and operated a fishing resort. Once out of high school I tried a couple of semesters of college, only to quit halfway through the Spring term; I decided at that time that college wasn't for me.

Then I decided to follow my father's previous occupation as an auto mechanic. I graduated from a two-year of vocational training course and worked as a mechanic for five years. While in vocational training, I decided to join the National Guard where I eventually ended up working full-time for 32 years.

So how does all of this relate to writing? In one of my leadership schools, the instructor, who was an English teacher at a juvenile detention center, presented writing to me in a whole new way - a way that started to develop my interest in working with words.

I eventually went back to college on the GI Bill while I was working and earned my Bachelor's degree in Business Administration. Taking a class or two per semester at night and on weekends took me seven years to complete my degree.

Fast forward about 40 years and I now have published over 75 books on Amazon for Kindle, CreateSpace and other publishing platforms.

Besides my own writing, I also ghostwrite ebooks, books, reports, articles, blogs and do Kindle conversions for clients on a variety of topics.

Today my wife and I are retired from our careers and live in Gold Canyon, AZ. I now write as a retirement business where you'll find me happily sitting in my office typing away on my laptop as I work on my next book or ghostwriting project . . . that is if we are not traveling on a cruise ship - our new-found mode of travel.

www.ingramcontent.com/pod-product-compliance
Lightning Source LLC
Chambersburg PA
CBHW050810290526
45792CB00001B/57